Diabetes Your Way

A Guide to Success

Michelle Dart, MSN, PNP, CDE

Ringo Publishing, Inc.

Edited by Miranda L. Pennock

Ringo Publishing, Inc.

Cover photo © Sergej Khackimullin - Fotolia.com

ISBN-10:1479243167

ISBN-13: 971479243167

The information in this book is not intended to serve as a substitute for a physician, nurse practitioner or other healthcare provider or provide medical advice. The author does not intend to give medical advice contrary to that of an attending physician. The reader should contact their physician for specific concerns about their health status or prior to making any changes in their healthcare regimen.

DEDICATION

This book is dedicated to my father who lives with Type 2 Diabetes. Thank you, Dad for always believing in me and standing beside me along this journey. You inspire me. I have learned so much from you, not only about diabetes, but life and how important it is to have a parachute with me.

I also want to dedicate this to my son, Richard, who lives with Type 1 Diabetes. I am very proud of you. You help me to see that everyone is unique and your diabetes is not going to always follow the books. I hope you always find a way to live life with diabetes your way.

Thank you to my family and friends who have supported and empowered me. Most of all, to my husband, Rick, I want to thank you for always believing in me, even if I wasn't so sure of myself. Thank you for pushing me to reach for my dreams and being right there beside me. Hunter and Cobra, you are my shining stars and make me want to be a better person.

I also want to thank Miranda for editing this book. I look forward to working on many more with you.

Diabetes Your Way
Table of Contents

Michelle A. Dart

Introduction

Welcome to life with Diabetes. You may have picked up this book because you have Type 1 or Type 2 Diabetes, you have a parent or child with diabetes, or you are a support person to someone who has diabetes. You may even be a health care provider who wants to know if this book is worth recommending to a patient. You are part of the majority of the population. Regardless of the reason, this book will hopefully be an inspiration to live happy, healthy lives with diabetes.

I do not claim to have all the answers. There is no promise for a cure in the last few pages, or any pages of this book for that matter. There isn't one single answer that is going to help everyone struggling with diabetes. We are all unique. Our bodies are different. Our lifestyles vary. Our values and goals are not exactly the same as the next person's. We are individuals with our very own life with diabetes.

Whoever said "keep it simple" did not know what life with diabetes is like. A more realistic goal is to "keep it as simple as possible". If anyone told you this would be an easy journey, they were wrong. Anything that is worthwhile in life is rarely simple, yet nothing is impossible. You have the tools within you to have an amazing life with diabetes — you may not even realize what you have, but you will learn more as you create your life with diabetes.

It doesn't matter if you have the top endocrinologist, the best diabetes educator or the strongest support system. These are all helpful, but do not guarantee successful diabetes management. The words in this book will not offer any more than a source of inspiration and motivation. What matters is what you choose to do with what you have. This book isn't designed to be a main source of diabetes education. There are great educational resources in Chapter 11. Take advantage of every aspect of your support system. Your

provider and educator can help you determine particular

patterns created by your lifestyle.

There really isn't a nutrition plan, exercise plan or

diabetes management plan that is made for everyone. Diabetes

is not "one size fits all." There are guidelines that sometimes

are vague or may seem too strict. It is all in your perception.

Diabetes self-management means the person with diabetes makes

their own management decisions. This DOES NOT replace

proper medical management. Your health care provider helps

to guide the medical management, but the follow through and

decisions made at home are your responsibility. Diabetes

education is a very important part of daily management.

Intelligent decisions are made when we not only find the

information we need, but fully understand it. Don't be

afraid to ask for more information. Successful

self-management starts with knowledge about diabetes, self-

awareness, increased self-confidence, little fear and, of course,

a safety net.

Specific instructions and detailed maps will not always

work. I will not tell you what you need to do; I respect that you

have thoughts and ideas of your own. I trust you know what

has and hasn't worked when you have tried different routines.

You have to be comfortable with your routine in order for it to

be successful. Throughout this book, you will find starting

points to create your diabetes life path. Only you know you

best. Personalize your own management plan.

As you read through "Diabetes Your Way," you will

learn some helpful ideas to make your daily diabetes management

as unique as you are. There are no perfect answers, but what I

hope you will find in this book is empowerment to live the life

you want to live and how to successfully self-manage your

your diabetes. I hope you find the creativity to make diabetes

fit into your lifestyle. If you can't embrace it, then find a way

to change it. Creating a life with diabetes is challenging, but

not impossible.

Enjoy your journey.

Michelle A. Dart

Important Note

Choosing to not take care of your diabetes puts you at risk for serious complications, hospitalization and death. This writer does not support any medical management that is not approved by the individual's physician. Encouragement to manage diabetes in a way that fits one's lifestyle is not meant to take the place of having open and honest conversations with healthcare providers and making decisions together regarding blood glucose monitoring, oral medications or insulin dosage and delivery. Our healthcare providers are not able to help us make the best decisions for us when they do not have all the information about how we manage diabetes day to day. Please contact your provider before implementing any changes in your routine that may impact your diabetes control.

Michelle A. Dart

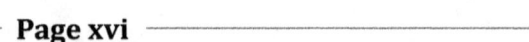

Chapter 1 — You've Got to Own It!

It's true. You have to own it to change it ... to perfect it. If

you haven't accepted your diagnosis of diabetes, then you

may not be ready to take on this journey. Here are a few

questions to consider:

- ☐ Do you have diabetes? If the answer is yes, this book is
  for you! If the answer is no, continue to the next
  question.

- ☐ Does your child/parent/loved one have diabetes?
  If the answer is yes, this book is for you! If the
  answer is no, continue to the next question.

- ☐ Do you feel you have a good understanding about
  how diabetes works? If the answer is yes, this book is
  for you! If the answer is no, this book is for you,

Michelle A. Dart

in addition to a strong recommendation to work with your diabetes educator.

- ☐ Do you work hard to manage diabetes or support someone in their diabetes management? If the answer is no, this might be a good time to get involved, learn more with a diabetes educator and read this book for inspiration.

- ☐ Do you get frustrated with blood sugars and lab results despite significant efforts to improve? If the answer is yes, this book is for you! If the answer is no, is it because things are going well and you are content? That is great! If the answer is no because you haven't been making many efforts to improve your diabetes management, I would invite you to read this book and let me know if you were inspired in any way to live healthier and happier with diabetes.

If you are ready, we will move on to owning our diabetes.

Owning it means we accept it. Good, bad, or indifferent, it's

reality. If you ignore it, it becomes a bigger monster to

face. Acceptance does not mean you have to love it! We often

accept concepts in our minds before we act. The process

between acceptance and action is different for everyone. Some

people are propelled into action as soon as they accept the

idea. Other people need to process and plan, taking more

time. One way is not any better than the other.

This is a process that takes time. Not everyone is ready to jump

into an unanticipated life with diabetes. There are times that

someone will take the medication the doctor orders and

doesn't understand what it is for or even that they have a

diagnosis of diabetes. We can't fix something we don't

realize is broken. Healthcare providers are often rushed in

appointments and we miss bits and pieces when they

talk fast or we feel their urgency to get through the visit. We live in an era that requires us to ask questions. Seek information about what diagnoses you have, when blood work will be drawn and what will be tested, and when your next appointment will be. If you have more specific questions, keep a running list of them and highlight the most important ones to focus on in case you run out of time in the visit.

With education, comes a sense of ownership. Ask questions, read and if you have Internet access or a local library, do some research. Often we become emotionally invested. This is one way to spark motivation. Or, this could reinforce denial. Information is not always accurate. If you aren't sure what reliable resources there are, see Chapter 11 for some valid resources.

You may have already incorporated diabetes self-management into your routine. Even if you have embraced it and dedicate a lot of time and energy into your diabetes management, you may be feeling as though you are missing something. It's called a life. Your routine may be so regimented and you crave information about the blood sugar numbers and react to every reading, trying so hard to keep those numbers in a certain range that you forget to enjoy life. You should be praised for all of your efforts. Owning diabetes is important, but it can easily become a source of obsession.

We let numbers define us. **"Grown-ups love figures. When you tell them that you have made a new friend, they never ask you any questions about essential matters. They never say to you, 'what does his voice sound like? What games does he love best? Does he collect butterflies?'**
Instead, they demand: 'how old is he? How many brothers has he? How much does he weigh? How much money does his father make?'

Only from these figures do they think they have

learned anything about him." – The Little Prince

And for many people, the often heard question is, "what is

your blood sugar?" The blood sugar reading is a reflection

of our actions, but we often forget there are outside forces that

impact our readings, as well. We can't control hormonal

surges, illness, injuries, sleep disruptions or the things that

trigger us to feel stressed. We must take care of our bodies and

our diabetes, but at the same time recognize there can be other

factors involved in changes that occur.

I agree that more information is very helpful in determining

patterns to decide what is working and what isn't working.

Can there be too much information? Yes, actually there can.

Technology allows us the ability to get frequent information

from continuous glucose monitors. Insulin pumps are

amazing because we can take things into consideration such

as the amount of insulin previously administered, the time of insulin administration, and the ability to change the amount of basal insulin even temporarily. We can also factor in how much active insulin is impacting the current blood sugar. This much information is great, but can also be overwhelming. These tools are meant to help fine tune management for each individual based on their needs.

There is a fine line between being focused and being obsessed with our diabetes. Compare this with someone who is trying so hard to lose weight. That number on the scale is important to us, just like the number on the glucose meter is important. It's easy to think, "I did something to affect the number" and to want to check it repeatedly. And we hold ourselves responsible for the number that appears. We base our value on that number. What a roller coaster ride!

Owning it doesn't mean we have to be so driven, yet taking ownership can be a strong motivator. Learn from others who take those numbers, make sense of them and make educated decisions based on that information. Make those numbers useful to you and be sure they aren't working against you.

Sometimes it is just easier to let someone instruct us on the tasks we need to do and not necessarily understand why. A provider who can address your diabetes isn't really negotiable. Whether you have a primary care provider or an endocrinologist, it is important to have them on your team, but you are the captain. Have your provider explain why they recommend one thing over another. Be honest about anything that prevents you from following their recommendations, even if it is as simple as you found something that works just as well and fits into your day. Our resources are not nearly as helpful if they aren't appropriate for our current lifestyle. Your provider may be able to help you come up with other options if they know something is not working well. If your provider doesn't listen to you, it is time to find another provider. It is helpful to have a provider you can express your thoughts and ideas with openly and honestly while trusting their knowledge and taking their ideas into consideration.   You are the leader of the team and get

the final call.

Chapter 2 — Examining Your Life

You are unique. Your experiences, personality, temperament, values and beliefs are different from everyone else. How can diabetes management possibly be the same for everyone? We know the basics of diabetes self-management from years of research. Healthcare providers have a vast amount of knowledge and skills to help you be successful. Being able to communicate questions and concerns to your provider will open up doors to discussions that will help you further examine how best to manage your diabetes.

Chances are you already have a bit of knowledge about diabetes and may even be an expert. In fact, you are the expert. Only you know your body best and how you respond to different issues that affect your blood sugar and overall level of diabetes control.

Control … this is interesting to me. Who or what is in control? Seriously, think about your day from the moment you get up. If you could spend your day without regard to managing your diabetes, how would you want your day to look? Can you make adjustments in your diabetes routine to spend your days the way you want to?

Some people need that routine because they feel their blood sugar is less "controlled" if there are fluctuations in their schedule. They feel like they are restricted or tied down to the diabetes management. Again, who or what is in control? Don't despair; there are tips in chapter four to help you make changes in your routine, if necessary.

There are many aspects of our lives that become routine or ritualistic. Without giving any thought to our actions, we proceed through our days having performed numerous activities. To really examine your life, you need to make a conscious effort to learn what your patterns are. Some of your actions do not have a significant impact on your diabetes or overall health. Focusing on those areas that influence your diabetes self-management will be helpful as you create a life with diabetes that you can live with.

Keeping a journal about your daily routine can give insight to how you are really benefitting or negatively affecting your diabetes management. It can be difficult to maintain a journal for a length of time. If you find you do well journaling for a day or two and then the record keeping declines, then plan to do two days at a time and then repeat every few days. Patterns can be detected with less than a week of journal records.

How do you recognize patterns? I like to see something that is consistent for more than two days in a row or >50% of the time. For example, you may realize that you exercise more on certain days and when you compare your blood glucose records, you see a pattern of higher blood glucose on days when you haven't exercised. There are more factors than exercise alone that play into this, but I would question how you feel on those days after the elevated blood glucose. Getting better control over the blood glucose may help you feel better, resulting in more activity.

While a journal may be helpful, if journaling isn't for you, there are other options. A journal may give you information about a variety of things such as, eating patterns, exercise routines and if there are any areas that can be improved. Calendars can be very helpful to put some notes on to help you remember changes in the routine or reminders. A bulletin board or refrigerator may be a great place to keep a recording system. Most blood glucose meters have an easily accessible memory and this lends to writing out fewer records. This is great, but doesn't give you the visual that makes patterns stand out. If you have the supplies and ability to download the information onto a computer, it's even better. But at least once a week, going through the memory and writing down the readings can be helpful.

If you are already aware of a specific target area that you know isn't working with your goals, starting here is another approach. Consider what actions you take that can influence this goal. The actions we don't take can also have an impact. Ask yourself if there is one thing you can do today that would be a positive step in that direction.

Share with me your goals. Share your goals with someone, anyone you can open up to. Share your goals with yourself. Write them down and put them in a special container that holds your goals safely until you accomplish them. There is no better way to be accountable than to make it real. Once you speak of your goal, it becomes real. You can almost touch it. And the more often you speak of it, the bigger it grows and you can feel the excitement build.

It is like planting a garden. Each thought is a seed. Every time you talk about your goal, you are watering the seed. Share your story often. Just as your garden needs frequent attention, so does your goal. Unless you take that seed, put it in the ground and water it, it will simply stay a seed. You can even plant it, but leave it unattended and it will remain a seed. How do you want to handle your goals? Are you ready to tend to your own garden? You can wait for someone to bring you flowers, or you can plant your own and design the garden your way.

One of my favorite, most inspirational poems is

"Comes the Dawn,"

by Veronica A. Shoffstall.

After a while you learn the subtle difference

Between holding a hand and chaining a soul,

And you learn that love doesn't mean leaning

And company doesn't mean security,

And you begin to learn that kisses aren't contracts

And presents aren't promises,

And you begin to accept your defeats

Diabetes Your Way

With your head up and your eyes open

With the grace of a woman, not the grief of a child,

And you learn to build all your roads on today,

Because tomorrow's ground is too uncertain for

plans,

And futures have a way of falling down in mid-flight.

After a while you learn

That even sunshine burns if you get too much.

So you plant your own garden and decorate your own

soul,

Instead of waiting for someone to bring you flowers.

And you learn that you really can endure...

That you really are strong,

And you really do have worth.

And you learn and learn... With

every goodbye you learn.

This is your life ... your garden ... your diabetes. Don't be afraid to toss that first seed in the ground. Set a goal and go after it. Don't expect your garden to look like anyone else's garden. The experience of diabetes is yours alone. There is not another person whose life is just like yours, has the same diabetes characteristics or reactions to stress or medications. Your providers experience with your diabetes is not your experience. They can only understand as much as you share with them. Sharing your goals will help others to understand what is important to you. Don't get me wrong. Your experience with diabetes may be yours alone, but this does not mean you have to be alone in your life with diabetes. Having a strong support system or people who may help you tend to your garden is important. Who is part of your support system? In what ways do you feel supported? What areas do you need more support on?

A support system can be made up of a variety of people including, family, friends, support groups, diabetes online community, community organizations and healthcare providers. Make a list of your support persons and how they support you. If anyone on

your list has a negative impact on your life, you may want to

consider ways to increase the positive influences on your life and

diabetes management. When you are motivated to make changes, you

need people who are supportive of you and want to help build you

up and not tear you down. Don't let your garden get overrun with

weeds.

Michelle A. Dart

Chapter 3 — Obstacles and Barriers

There are many obstacles that get in the way of achieving our goals. That is all they are ... bumps in the road. I see obstacles as the everyday annoyances that we face. They may or may not bother us. A barrier, on the other hand, is a wall that we hit and that is where we stay, unless we really want to make that effort to tear it down. Often times, the barriers are specific to us. What prevents me from doing a specific task? What keeps me from doing what I know I need to do to be healthy? Why don't I take back my life and live it in a healthy way that fits me and my lifestyle? This is where it is challenging. We each will have a different solution. We can't find all the answers in a book or online. Sometimes we have to be very creative.

There is always an option to overcome the various road blocks that slow us down, drag us around and make us want to just give up. But we don't have to give up. Honestly, we don't have to do anything. Understanding that there are consequences to every choice we make, some good and some not so good. We can choose to act or choose to stay right where we are.

Even if we choose not to change a thing, those barriers and obstacles will find us. Everyone has a battle to face and we are all equipped differently to handle these situations. One method of overcoming an obstacle may work great for you, but not someone else. There is always more than one way to approach things.

Your attitude toward obstacles and barriers will have an impact on how you act. If we feel the obstacle course is overwhelming, we can break it down into manageable pieces. If we hit a barrier that has us frustrated, sometimes it is best to step back and really look at what is before us. Determining what you need to overcome the barrier arms you for battle. Sometimes we don't know what we are really facing or make choices that prove not to be the best option for us. All of this has an effect on the outcome of your journey.

What about the consequences of our choices? How do we really know what they will be? Well, it is hard to predict. Again, we are all different in our approach. You can approach it armed with education and statistics. You may approach it with passion and motivation, driven by conscious decisions for what you feel is best for you. Or you may be easy going and comfortable going with the flow and facing each challenge as it comes your way.

Our approach may not even be the best for us. Examine your approach. You may try another approach and find it works better for you.

Educate yourself. Find out how your body and your blood sugar react to different foods and activities. Learn about long-term complications that can occur if diabetes is not managed well. Going forward without this information is frightening and full of risks. Falling down without having the tools to get back up can be challenging if not impossible. Safety nets are not for the weak, they are for the strong and determined.

Here are some examples of actions with potential consequences:

Action	Consequences
No Action	We stay right where we are. Diabetes can't improve without action of some sort, beyond what we are currently doing. Things can get worse, though. There is always a risk of complications or new issues arising when we don't give ourselves the attention we need.
"Healthy" Eating	A healthy body lends to a healthy mind. Feeling better impacts how we move forward and what

goals we may set for ourselves. Sometimes we feel so good that we wonder why we didn't eat better, sooner.

If we try to follow every "healthy" recommendation, there truly are very few foods left for us to choose from. If a diet is too restrictive, we can deny ourselves of important nutrients and even risk low blood glucose. Some of us feel very deprived. The risk of "cheating" is there and when we fall, we feel guilty. Sometimes the information we hear becomes overwhelming and then who knows what we can eat? Or we try to incorporate all of this knowledge into our routine and find it to be a daunting task when we really need to keep it simple.

"Unhealthy" Eating

Enjoyment of every bite and its taste often goes along with the less healthy foods. There is little nutritional value to help our bodies function and often has the ability to do damage to our bodies. Since we get little nutrition, we often are more hungry, we gain weight and have less control of our blood glucose. We may find more criticism from others. Some of us may already feel guilty because we are aware of the damage we can do by feeding ourselves these unhealthy choices.

"Balanced" Eating

Our bodies cannot survive on protein alone. There is a need for all of the food groups. By eating a balanced plate, we are providing our body with foods that will break down into blood glucose at different rates and improve our potential for successful diabetes control. We tend to feel healthier when we stick to a balanced diet and less deprived of foods we enjoy. With this method, we can work any food into our meal planning.

Having a balance also pertains to portion sizes. A "balanced" plate does not

	have double servings of the food options. Being aware of what foods are best to have more of when we do not feel satisfied is important to maintain the balance.
No Exercise	We are unable to reap the benefits of exercise to our physical and emotional well being. The reason for no exercise is important to consider. If it is beyond our physical limitations, that means we do not have a choice to perform the exercise. In this case, a physical therapist may be a good option. It is not likely that a person has no activity at all if there isn't a physical disability.
Limited Exercise	First of all, some activity is better than no activity. It doesn't matter how we get the activity; every movement counts. Again there may be physical limitations to prevent a very active lifestyle. In this case, our bodies lack the benefits of deep breathing, increased

	heart pumping and overall energy. Physical therapy may be the source of activity. Stretching even counts as an activity.
	Maybe we choose not to be active. Mentally, we can limit ourselves. When this happens, we are giving ourselves less than what our bodies deserve and miss out on the emotional benefits of routine exercise.
Moderate Exercise	Your body will benefit from a moderate exercise routine. The only negative consequences would be the risk of injury. Some may say they miss out on time they need for other things and see this as a negative consequence. Yet, exercise often results in increased energy to accomplish those other things in life.
Intense Exercise	This level of exercise can be great for your heart and overall well-being. There is an increased risk for injury. There may be improved

	diabetes control or we can find that the ups and downs of our blood sugar are unpredictable, making it harder to manage. Even with the health benefits of this level of exercise, there is a risk of high blood sugars from adrenaline. When the adrenaline comes down, so will the blood sugar. The rise is only temporary. The effects of exercise on our overall health, outweighs the short~lived elevated blood glucose. *Some may find the high blood sugars last longer and need to be treated. Talk this over with your healthcare provider. **Always discuss with your provider any changes you would like to make in your physical activity prior to starting a new routine.
Medication Not Taken as Prescribed	One consequence is the missed opportunity for anticipated results from medication. At the same time, we avoid side effects from these medications that can lead to additional issues. Risks and benefits should be carefully weighed when choosing not to take medication.

	Sometimes it is not a choice and we can't take the medication because of side effects. Financially, medication puts a strain on most of our wallets. Making a choice between having a place to live and taking medication is a reality. The consequences are the same, regardless if it is by choice or not. **see Chapter 11 Resource Guide for information on financial aspects of Diabetes care If side effects are an issue, discuss other options with your provider.
Medication Taken as Prescribed	Taking medication as prescribed can have the anticipated effects by managing symptoms. There is always a risk of side effects with any medication. There is also a risk of the medication interacting poorly with another medication, prescription and over the

	counter. When taken correctly, medication may be successful in managing diabetes.
Medication Self~ Management	This primarily is for those people treated with insulin by injection or the insulin pump. Oral medications should be adjusted only by your health care provider. Our provider should know all that we take, including over the counter medications that we self~ manage. People taking insulin injections can be highly independent in adjusting the doses based on food intake, blood glucose and activity level, among other factors. We know our bodies best and with our healthcare provider's guidance, we can learn to manage insulin doses according to our own bodies and our activity level, leading to better diabetes control.
Do Not Keep Routine Visits With Our Healthcare	There is unawareness of how well diabetes is

Providers (primary provider, endocrinologist, dentist, podiatrist, ophthalmologist, other specialties)	Controlled or overall health may be. We do not have to worry about bad news if we just don't go. We do not have to be told what to do or how to best manage our care. We also miss opportunities to see how we are doing and learn more information to improve our health. We deny ourselves a chance to get much of what we need to manage our own health. What we don't know can, in fact, hurt us. **see Chapter 11 Resource Guide for information on financial aspects of diabetes care
Keep Routine Visits With Our Healthcare Providers (primary provider, endocrinologist, dentist, podiatrist, ophthalmologist, other specialties)	We are more likely to learn about problems or potential problems before there is irreversible damage. This gives us the opportunity to make educated decisions about our healthcare. Yes, we may face difficult challenges and decisions. This can be emotionally stressful and it is difficult to confront fears, often of the unknown.

	As unappealing as it sounds, we gain a lot from this information. We get choices this way. Being educated about our health empowers us to choose how best to manage our diabetes and every other aspect of our health.
Do Not Have Lab Work Drawn (Hemoglobin A1c/Estimated Average Glucose)	This avoids any needles, discomfort and bruising. Again, what we don't know can hurt us. Without this information, we make decisions that have the potential to be harmful. If we don't understand the value of the information we can get from the lab work, we may not be as likely to follow up. By not having the lab work done, we also deny our healthcare providers this information. Lab work tells a story about us that can give insight into changes that can't be seen or heard. **see Chapter 11 Resource Guide for information on financial aspects of diabetes care

Have Lab Work Drawn	By obtaining this information, we arm ourselves and our providers with additional tools to improve our health. Knowing what we can and can't influence about our bodies can put us in the right direction to living a healthy way that we love.

This does not include every possible consequence. Just as we all are unique, consequences will vary and our response to those consequences will be different as well.

Chapter 4 — Change ... Really?

"Nobody can go back and start a new beginning, but anyone can start today and make a new ending."

-Maria Robinson

You may be saying, "I don't want to change!" and that's okay. Let's face it, forcing someone to make a change never works. Someone may tell us we need to eat specific foods because they are the healthy options. I know there are a number of things on that list that someone will say, "I don't eat that." Instead of looking at what is a good option or a bad option, why not make a check mark next to everything you like, regardless of where it is on the list? If you have more on the unhealthy list than the healthy list, what does that tell you?

There is a way to balance things out with portion sizes. You know what foods are healthy and you know what is junk food. If you choose to eat mostly junk food, the consequence is an unhealthy body, elevated blood sugar and long term complications. I believe even the pickiest eater can find a way to benefit from their nutrition. Everything is a balance. You may not want to change your lifestyle today or even in the future, but what you can do, is make your lifestyle work for you. Work hard on the positive things you do for yourself as they become habit. Educate yourself so you understand the consequences of your choices to help you make decisions that are best for you.

You may also be thinking, "Why should I change?" That is a good question. You feel fine, the doctor hasn't told you there are any problems, yet you have Type 1 or Type 2 diabetes. So, why should you change? Ask yourself if you are more proactive or reactive?

Being proactive is saying you want to prevent the negative things you know have a potential to impact your life. By being reactive, you wait until there is any obvious issue impacting your life. How do you typically handle other things in your life besides diabetes?

The proactive thinker is looking ahead and knows there are some walls waiting that can hold us back from living independently. We know we always want an option to have a choice. We don't want to be faced with an unavoidable outcome, such as a stroke, heart attack or amputation. We understand the reality of life if we don't take action now. We are the worriers.

The reactive thinker often sees life as predetermined, out of our hands and we can't change what is meant to be.

So, why stress now over something that is inevitable? We don't feel we have control. Some feel a higher power makes all the choices for us. We strive to enjoy the here and now. We are more reckless in the care we take of our bodies. We know in the back of our mind what our future may hold for us. We also realize we can't predict what needs to be acted on or what is going to hold us back. I may focus on taking such good care of my diabetes and still get cancer. When we look back, can we say that we lived a life we loved?

One extreme or another is never a good thing. Again, we have to look for that balance. It is about making choices and compromises that are realistic to the way we live day to day.

Let's look at another perspective — "Why shouldn't you change?" Aaahhh. Even I get stuck on that one. I hesitate in my mind because I'm not really sure how I can rationally explain out loud why I don't want to or why it would not be a good option for me to make a change. Imagine someone asked you that question. What would your response be to changing the one thing you know you absolutely do not want to change or give up? Sometimes a little different perspective can impact how we view our life with diabetes.

You may be thinking, "I'm not convinced I even need to make a change." If we don't think there is a need for action, we aren't going to take action. In my fantasy world, everyone who is diagnosed with diabetes, regardless if it is Type 1 or Type 2, should receive in depth diabetes education. Maybe your doctor takes care of everything and you just do what you are told. Or you do part of what you are told and don't do some very important diabetes tasks. If you don't know how important it is to check your blood sugar, you aren't going to test as often as may be recommended. That blood sugar reading should be guiding you — not controlling you — but the number is useless if you don't fully understand what it is telling you.

Diabetes education is available. Your physician can do a referral for diabetes education. Your local support group is another source of education. A support group offers perspectives from people living with diabetes every day.

Connecting with this group of people is a great resource for "real life" living with diabetes. If no one offers you these options, ask about them. I can't stress enough how important it is to educate yourself about diabetes and all things that affect your life. It is difficult to determine what you need to know if you don't have a good enough idea of what you are expected to know.

"Your life does not get better by chance, it gets better by change."

**–Jim
Rohn**

Diabetes Your Way

Once we choose to make a change, we have to consider how to make that change. Change is not instantaneous. It is a process we go through. The starting point is not clear and it's hard to judge how well we are doing because the end is not always in sight. Here are some tips to help you through the process of change:

Ø Getting Started

- o Consider what it may take for you to get started

- o Consider what may have been holding you back from making the change

- o Make a plan

- o Set a date and stick to it!

- o Enlist a support person to help keep you motivated

☐ Keeping up the Momentum

- o Address obstacles as they come up

o Enjoy the little accomplishments that will lead you to your greatest accomplishment

o Call on your support system if you feel yourself slipping

o Keep the goal in sight as a reminder of where you are heading

Ø Finding the Finish Line

o Don't expect to see the checkered flag until you are right on top of it or even past it

o Remind yourself it could be beyond this last bump in the road

Whether you can see it or not, your goal is there, so don't give up!

"Courage doesn't always roar. Sometimes courage is the little voice at the end of the day that says I'll try again tomorrow."

-Mary Anne Radmacher

Michelle A. Dart

Chapter 5 — The You Factor

Diabetes is very overwhelming. There is a lot to know and understand. If it seems too overwhelming, see if you can visit with a certified diabetes educator. The educator can help you learn at your pace and focus on the areas that are most important to you. As an educator, I would have you look at your daily routine before making changes. Why change something that is working well? Keeping written records of blood sugar, medication, activity and nutrition can be extremely helpful in learning how diabetes can fit into that normal daily routine.

You may be feeling like you are expected to change who you are and how you live your life, asking "What about what I want?" First of all, no one can take anything from you that you aren't willing to give up. When you are in a discussion about how diabetes is best managed, you are hearing about recommended practices based on years of research. This is the education piece. This isn't about creating a new you.

It is about being who you are and creating a life that helps you

build on who you are to have a happy, successful diabetic life.

If you feel you are being pressured to do things, it is a result of

your interactions with your provider. Your providers are all

unique, just as you and your diabetes are unique. Initially, you

will get your first impression and that sets up preconceptions

about that provider and may keep you from feeling comfortable

throughout your relationship. First visits with a new provider

can be difficult because you are beginning a new relationship

and each need to get to know one another. An open mind is

important to get through the first few visits when you and the

provider both become more relaxed in your interaction. If you

can't find a comfort zone with your provider where you can

be open and honest, it is time to find a new provider. They can

be of the most benefit when you are honest about what you really

do day to day to manage your diabetes. And it is okay if you are

not perfect 100 percent of the time! You can have it your way, just remember every choice has a consequence. You have a right to participate in your diabetes management. The more you learn, the more you get comfortable managing your diabetes independently, the greater the opportunity to make safe choices for a healthy lifestyle that doesn't sacrifice who you are and how you enjoy life.

What holds you back from managing diabetes your way? Think about it. Think about all the things you could or should be doing to best manage your diabetes. Now take each one and write down two reasons why you don't find a way to make changes that you would like to make.

Maybe you feel limited because you don't have an insulin pump since your physician will not recommend one for you because they have criteria requiring you to test your blood sugar four times a day and you are only testing twice a day. (just an example) The reasons can be external and out of our personal control or something internal such as fear, anxiety, anger, etc. Your reasons will be individual to you.

I can think of several reasons not to do something and I'm sure I have heard "it sucks" a number of times when I asked this question. I agree. Diabetes sucks! It also is something that isn't going away. Hopefully technology will prove that statement wrong. My point is, if you have Type 1 Diabetes, you will always need insulin. It's just the delivery methods of insulin that are changing. If you have Type 2 Diabetes, you can become symptom free by losing weight, eating healthy, exercising and taking oral medication. You will always need to be aware that symptoms can come back if you gain weight. Sometimes aging triggers symptoms to return. And, even with the best control, there is the possibility insulin will be needed someday. It is always there; it is just controlled or uncontrolled.

Once you identify what is holding you back from living a life with diabetes that you want, the next step is coming up with a list of ideas for how to conquer each one. Whatever comes to your mind, write it down and come up with a couple ideas that may work for you. Every now and then we all need to check in with ourselves to see what is working and what is not. Remember, you can't change what isn't perceived to be broken.

Getting started can be one of the most difficult things to do. Keeping things up the way we want can be even more challenging. Do you postpone things and when you finally get to it, you fly right through it? Or do you come up with ideas and without really planning it out, just jump right in and fizzle out later down the road?

Knowing which you tend to do in other aspects of your life, as well as managing your diabetes, can be very important in helping you plan how to make it work best for you. Personally, I am a "postponer." I have been that way as long as I can remember. Does it always work? No, unfortunately, it doesn't. But that is when my creativity comes out ... when I am running on a deadline. With diabetes, those deadlines are either the ones we set for ourselves or when time runs out and we have this complication to deal with. This is a great example of, "I know what is best, but I do it this way because it works best for me." Have I been successful being a "postponer?" Yes, but it has its consequences as well.

I am also a "jumper." I come up with ideas that I am passionate about. I set goals for myself and will plan it right out. I jump on in. So, I don't always know exactly what I am getting myself in for and I hit roadblock after roadblock. I am so motivated that these little roadblocks are just that to me — little. I put all my energy and thoughts into the goal that I wear myself out with one challenge after another and I just don't have the energy for another obstacle in my way. Is all lost this way? Not really. All my hard work and focus may be useful for my next passion.

I like to think I'm "balanced." It sounds like the "diet soda cancels out the candy bar" statement. I'm not saying one approach is better than the other or that these are the only approaches. A good approach is to:

1.	Understand the problem; educate yourself.

2.	Self-assessment; find out what works and doesn't work within your routine.

3.	Look at what isn't working and be realistic as to whether this is something you care to change, understand enough about to change, and what, if anything, are you willing to sacrifice; discard it if you are absolute about not wanting to change your routine.

4.	Consider the consequences; discard the ones you are comfortable living with and re- evaluate the consequences that you are uneasy about.

5.   Examine what aspects of your daily routine are affected by the particular change; discard the ones you know you aren't willing to disrupt your routine for or set it aside as something to find a creative way to manage.

6.   What is left should be smaller, more manageable choices that you can set as your goal and be pretty confident you can be successful.

Understand that every change, no matter how insignificant it may seem, can change your whole future. Eating one healthy food choice a day versus all junk food is still an improvement. Moving your arms and/or legs for 10 extra minutes a day, like when you are watching television, is still an improvement over 10 less minutes of exercise. Every movement counts. Checking the blood sugar one time a day is better than never checking. We all have to start somewhere. Just don't expect yourself to go from inactivity to being consistent with a behavior change at your maximum potential right out of the gate. Remember what can happen if you are a "jumper." You will fizzle fast. Pace yourself. Rushing along and stumbling will not get you to your goal any faster.

What if it doesn't work? Nobody likes to set himself up for failure. The word failure means different things for different people. Failure can mean it just didn't work. Now we need to find another way to make it work. For some, failure is taken personally. To fail at something we work hard for can often lead to feeling as though we failed as a person and not just that our idea failed. Get rid of the word "fail." Some things work and some things don't. It is a part of life and often happens for a reason. You are the main factor in the equation. Add diabetes and life will never be dull.

Everything you add to the equation will impact your life. *Make it something good!*

Michelle A. Dart

Chapter 6 — If It is Broken, Fix it

Only you know when something is working for you or not. If you decide you aren't happy with a result or feel a need to make a change, it's broken. Once you make the decision to fix what's broken, you can start working on what you choose to bring you to that level of diabetes control you are comfortable with. If it doesn't seem broken to you, there isn't much you can fix.

If something isn't working, it isn't meant to and it is often a sign that we need to try something different. Take something as simple as trying a new exercise plan to help you lose weight. Two weeks later you haven't lost a pound. That's upsetting, but it's not all your fault. You tried and it didn't work. Take joy in the fact you didn't gain any weight. Results aren't automatic. If we try one thing and it doesn't seem to be working, we either need to try something different or add something we can do that gives us an added boost to reach our goals. Don't be so quick to give up on yourself. You have more strength than you realize and you will get there. You may stumble and you may fall, but there is always an option to get back up.

What about "I know I should, but...?" We accept that something needs to change and we fully understand how it would benefit us, but there is something that holds us back. Here is where we exercise the right to say, "I don't want to change." Let's look at those things you know you don't want to change. Maybe you have valid reasons something should NOT change.

If there is a benefit to continue with your current lifestyle, you will not have an interest in changing it. One way to really know if it is worth changing is to look at the pros and cons. Say, I test my blood sugar twice a day instead of four times a day like my doctor recommended. It is working well for me and my blood sugars look great to me.

Diabetes Your Way

Consider the potential outcomes of continuing to test only twice a day:

1.   I only see that one moment in time when I see the number on the meter. I can only do so much with that information.

2.   A blood sugar can fluctuate greatly throughout the day. I am limiting myself by not getting information about how my body responds to food, exercise and my overall schedule.

3.   I have to consider that my blood sugar can be much higher, contributing to long term complications and I can't fix it if I don't have enough information.

4.   I could suffer significant low blood sugars if my blood sugar is typically lower right before dinner and then I eat much later than usual.

If I knew my patterns, I would have known to

have a snack to avoid the low blood sugar.

This is just an example of possible outcomes, but could be a much

longer list with serious, life-threatening consequences.

Examining what should stay the same in our routine means we

really need to understand the consequences of what we choose to

do or choose not to do. Consequences are not necessarily going

to be obvious right away, but how we live today will always

impact our tomorrow.

If something is broken, is it always worth fixing? When it

comes to your life, yes, it is worth fixing. You need to see your

worth to be willing to make the effort to fix something broken

in your life. What tools do you have?

You always have your inner strength and willpower. Some days

it may feel like there is not enough strength to keep up the

fight against diabetes. It is there, even if it doesn't feel that way. What other challenges have you overcome? How do you typically approach an area in your life that is "broken?" What you need to survive day after day is within you.

Leaving something broken until something else breaks and the next thing falls apart just adds to feeling overwhelmed. It is much easier to fix one thing than to look at several things that are broken. How do we know where to start? Keep it simple and work on issues one at a time. Break it down into manageable pieces.

If you are going to fix it, fix it right the first time. Life is short. We don't want to keep working on the same issues all the time. If an issue keeps coming up, that tells us we need a better solution, something that can last. Be realistic about what you can and will do. If you know you will not be able to follow through on something, there is no need to include it in your plan. The problem will just keep coming back.

To fix it the right way, it may mean extra effort or more time invested. It may be well worth it if it helps solve the problem. Some people prefer quick fixes, but too often we have to fix it again and again. What would you do with the free time when you have solved a problem and don't need to address that problem again? If we don't spend our days chasing down the problems and fixing them, we can actually enjoy life. Not addressing the problems can leave you feeling overloaded as problems build one on top of another until we are unable to see a way out.

Some people follow the belief that if they put as much effort into some things, they will set themselves up for the opportunity to stop and enjoy life once in awhile. Other people allow problems to build and become so overwhelming they are left frozen. All is not lost. Take advantage of that time standing still and take a deep breath. It may be a great opportunity to really look at the big picture of what needs to be dealt with. It is so easy to get focused on the little things and lose sight of the big picture.

Waiting to fix something that is broken can lead to even more damage, making the task even more daunting. It's easier to fix a slow leak in a pipe than to fix a geyser! The power of the impact on our lives grows like the weeds in our garden. The choice is yours. Which would you prefer?

Michelle A. Dart

Chapter 7 ~ The Road Less Traveled

"People travel to wonder at the height of mountains, at the huge waves of the sea, at the long courses of rivers, at the vast compass of the ocean, at the circular motion of the stars; and they pass by themselves without wondering."

– St. Augustine

Take a personal "road trip." Don't be afraid to step outside your comfort zone. Anticipate the many winding roads, hills and valleys with unpredictable curves along the way.

Consider where you are at in your journey. Maybe you are on a straight path where things are going well. You are content and not really looking to change. That is okay.

Sometimes simplicity is best. Maybe you are at the bottom of a mountain, facing a great challenge. Don't be afraid of what is before you, but anticipate the journey and how it will feel when you get to the top. Perhaps you are already at the top of the mountain and feeling accomplished. What is next? Stop and enjoy the view. Consider that next challenge you are preparing to take on. Feeling empowered can give us the momentum to take on something new.

On your travels, you may come to a lake or an ocean. Just as the vast water that ebbs and flows, we take the good with the bad. Jump in! The options are to sink or swim. If we sink, we are not failures. This just means we need a life preserver. We all need a little help sometimes. We need strength to swim ... courage to take the plunge. Where does this strength come from? It comes from within. It is there even when we feel we have little or no strength left. Others tell us we are stronger than we believe, but it is difficult to see it in ourselves. Think of another time where you felt your strength had been shaken and how you got through. You may not have felt strong during the process, but looking back, you had the strength to survive a difficult

challenge.

Often times, we find ourselves in the midst of a forest. We lose

direction and don't know where to go. We aren't sure who

or what to trust. There is fear of the unknown and the challenge

to find the right path is difficult. How do we make sense of it

all? For some, this is an adventure, yet others look for a safe place

to hide.

How do you approach the trip ahead? With fear? With

excitement? With dread? If the approach you have been using

isn't working, it may be time to look into new tactics.

Knowing how you approach life and its many forks in the road

is important. Do you typically stand there contemplating and

planning? Do you weigh all the pros and cons? Maybe you

move forward based on instinct? Whatever your approach,

you can make it work for you.

What do you pack for your road trip? I like to have something tangible to remember my trips. Writing about experiences, taking pictures, creating mementos can help provide inspiration for the next trip. Safety gear should always be on hand. That could be whatever will help you survive. I'm not referring to the basic needs of life, such as food, water, shelter, insulin, blood glucose monitor and the like — I'm talking about what will help you physically, emotionally and spiritually. This is different for each of us.

Anticipate that you will find empowerment along the road. One small step can take us for miles, but how far we travel is up to each one of us. Fear debilitates us. It makes us stop in our tracks and we miss many opportunities. Fear can also motivate us. We can refuse to let fear hold us back from something we really desire. If we let fear keep us from living, how can we move forward?

Something more significant than fear is the answer.

What is that for you? Do you want to prove something to yourself? Do you feel motivated because your family loves you and wants you to be healthy? Perhaps you thrive on the adrenaline that comes with that moment of accomplishment. Consider what is on the other side of that fear.

I have a fear of heights. Yet that doesn't stop me from reaching outside of my boundaries at times. What are your boundaries? How far can you go before you hit your limits? Remember you can always stretch your limits as you create the boundaries within which you live your life.

"It is not because things are difficult that we do not dare; it is because we do not dare that they are difficult." - Seneca

Creating a path of your own gives you freedom to take different turns along the way. We are in an environment that encourages us to be adventurous. We make a path that works for us and choose not to take the highway traveled by so many others.

Yes, we can learn from the experiences of others when we share a path, but we're more likely to go farther by taking our own path.

The choice is there. It is okay to follow the highway and travel with thousands of others, but this may not be the lifestyle you want to live. It is more difficult to follow another who created a path that has been beaten down by all the other travelers who have passed this way. There is not as much room for flexibility.

When you create a path of your own, the possibilities are endless. Your diabetes management can be tailored to your lifestyle. You have the power to imagine and bring your dreams to life. Don't spend time worrying that others will say you are wrong or you are not making the "right" decisions — there is no strict "right" or "wrong." What you do have is the potential for decisions to be "right" or "wrong" for you. Remember, though, just because it is not right for one, doesn't make it wrong for another person.

There is no room for judgment when we choose our path.

If someone doesn't support your chosen path, they are not needed on your team. Surround yourself with supporters, motivators and those who inspire you. Take advantage of all the things that provide inspiration. Does having diabetes inspire you to live differently? Does it inspire you to find a way to successful management, even if it isn't standard textbook management? Real life diabetes self- management often has some aspect of creativity and finding the way along unmarked paths.

Michelle A. Dart

Chapter 8 — Ready or Not!

How ready you are to make a change is another issue to consider. If you are ready, you will typically seek resources to help you accomplish your goal. If you are not ready, you will continue on with life as it is. Many of us teeter in between the two. We want it, but aren't quite ready to make that next move. Or, we know we need to make a change, but don't really want to change. What is holding you back? Let's look at a readiness scale. On this scale, we are not ready at level 1, but we are ready at a level 10.

How Ready Are You to...

Change an aspect of diabetes management; change eating patterns; change activity routine; change your perspective about life with diabetes; live the life you can

love, despite living with diabetes?

1	2	3	4	5	6	7	8	9	10

Level 1- not ready at all

Level 2/3- not completely against making a change, but not looking to make a change

Level 4/5/6- contemplating change

Level 8/9- seeing the positive in change and possibly taking steps toward change

Level 10- ready to make that change

Ask yourself these questions:

- What prevents me from being one step closer?

(*Why a level 5 and not a 7?)

- What put me this high up on the scale? (*Why a

level 6 and not a 4?)

What will it take for you to get one step closer? Consider what needs to change in order for you to get where you want to be. This will be different for everyone. Some people already know what is holding them back and can answer the question immediately. Often we need time to process it in our mind before we come up with an answer or idea of how to move forward.

Prepare yourself with more than one idea to approach an issue. When we go into something with one plan, and nothing to back it up, and something goes wrong, we are halted dead in our tracks. Now what? Make yourself a parachute of ideas. You can be moving right along and hit a bump in the road and that parachute of ideas may be the one thing to keep you going without much hesitation. This doesn't mean we will be prepared for every situation, but it's harder to stay down once we fall. Keep your feet off the ground and you will stay motivated.

Set yourself up for success, not failure. You want to be able to confidently take the next step. Confidence comes with knowledge, planning and drive. Without action, you stay right where you are. You can do it if you put your mind to it. If your mind is in other places, try to carve out a little bit of time to focus on you and your diabetes.

Maybe you are "just about ready to..." make a change, but something is holding you back. The only way to move forward is to figure out what it is that is keeping you from making changes. Previous experience shapes who we are and contributes to the choices we make. This is great if we can use it to our advantage. Consider the experiences that contribute in a positive way and how it can benefit you now. Will any of those experiences help you get where you want to be?

Negative experiences are just as important. We can learn as much from these as we can from the positive experiences. What did you learn from those experiences and how can that knowledge help you now? Gather all of the information together and add what is useful to your personal diabetes toolbox.

Sometimes we learn best by those negative aspects because we do

not want to repeat it. These patterns will continue to repeat as

long as we choose not to change anything.

When we take a step to avoid one of these lessons we have learned,

there are consequences. Everything is connected. For example,

maybe there is a change in insulin dosing, but there is no active

change in diet or exercise. Improving blood glucose with the

appropriate insulin dose can have an impact on those other areas.

The right amount of insulin allows us to use the food we are eating

and we may be less hungry. Changing the insulin dose, resulting in

improved blood sugar, can also spark more energy for exercise.

It's all connected.

It is not necessarily all about one single change. It is also about

being ready for how the change we are striving for may impact

other areas of our life. Being open and ready for the unexpected

will be important. Diabetes is an unexpected event in life for those who have been affected. Good or bad, life is full of the unexpected and unanticipated. How we respond to these surprises will shape how it impacts our life.

How can we possibly be ready for what we can't anticipate? We can be ready with the tools to face anything. One tool is flexibility. If we live a regimented lifestyle, it is difficult to be flexible. Any disruption in our routine can be very distressing and cause anxiety. Some anxiety can be productive and propel us into action to create stability again. But, some anxiety keeps us from going anywhere, which is counter-productive. Anxiety and depression should be evaluated by a healthcare provider if it is interfering with your life or keeping you from living the life you want. Anxiety is common and can be treated.

Another tool that can be found in a properly stocked toolbox is stress relief. We can't get through life without some stress. It is just impossible. Like anxiety, stress can motivate us or keep us in one place. How we deal with stress is up to us. It is important to have a plan. Some methods are healthy and others are not so healthy. Look at what has worked in the past to combat stress. Maybe it was an activity that provided distraction. Possibly it was some relaxation method, such as yoga or meditation. It may have even been addressing the issue head on.

Letting concerns over issues brew within our minds will only increase stress and anxiety. Facing the issues can put our minds at ease because there is less wondering about the outcome. Consider the consequences of your methods.

The third tool in our toolbox should be resilience. Resilience is that inner strength that helps us survive the tough times. This is when we are on automatic pilot. We do what needs to be done without having time to consider if stress or anxiety will interfere. We act without careful consideration, but in survival mode. We can stand up to the strongest storms, but we doubt ourselves when we face change or make decisions we know will have a strong impact on our lives.

The fourth tool that belongs in everyone's tool box is a desire to successfully manage diabetes and maintain the current lifestyle with as little disruption as possible. You have to want it to make it happen. Consider how passionate you are about creating a life you love while managing diabetes successfully. Is your passion strong enough to overcome the many challenges along the way? If you don't feel passionate now, look for what you can be passionate about while still having the ability to accomplish your goals.

There may be a variety of other tools that you like to have in your toolbox. Flexibility, stress management, resilience and desire are the basis for the toolbox that will help you reach your goals. You can add anything to your toolbox because it is yours.

Michelle A. Dart

Chapter 9 — Get Creative!

Think outside your diabetes toolbox. How can you take what you want and what you need to make it your own? Consider what is going on in your life. Do you live alone? Do you live on a limited income? Do you have your own family to support? Are you a full-time caregiver to someone with a disability? Do you have unlimited resources? Have you had a recent loss or significant change in your life? Do you have disabilities that limit your activity? Is diabetes a priority or are there more pressing issues today? What is your daily routine? What time does your day start and end? What in your routine is more important than spending a little time on you and your diabetes? Is diabetes your main focus? Does it interfere with you living a "normal" life? I still don't know a good definition for normal and leave it up to you to determine what is normal for you.

Every person with diabetes should have at least some of the

following basic management tools in their Diabetes Toolbox:

- Glucometer

- Test strips

- Lancets

- Syringes (Type 1 or Type 2)

- Insulin (Type 1 or Type 2)

- Extra pump supplies — battery, tubing, insertion kits, long acting insulin, contact number for pump company and diabetes educator/provider (Type 1 or Type 2)

- Oral medication (Type 2 only)

- Glucose tablets/gel

- Glucagon (if on insulin)

- Ketone urine test strips/meter (Type 1, occasionally Type 2)

- Juice and snack (example: peanut butter crackers, granola bar, small boxes of cereal)

- Medic alert identification tag (specify if taking insulin or metformin)

- Medication list

- Important contact numbers — ICE (in case of emergency) on cell

  phone, written list of emergency contact, physician contact,

  employer contact and anyone who may need to be called if you

  have an emergency situation

As you can see, some things can be used regardless of which

type of diabetes you have. Many of these tools will be the

same for everyone. There is no creative thinking involved in

the basics.

What can you add to the toolbox that will personalize it just for

you? Is there something you always rely on to get you or your

blood sugar back on track? Your toolbox can be as big as you need

it to be. Add to it. When you find something that helps you with

the rough spots, add it to your box.

As in the previous chapter, tools do not have to be something we

can touch or pick up with our hands. Make a list of everyone and everything that helps you live with diabetes. This can be anyone that is emotionally supportive of us, like family or friends. It can also be the inspiration we find in different activities and people. We can add our inner spirit and drive to move forward to our box.

What happens when we have used all of our tools and nothing is left in the box? That's when we get creative. It would be nice if we could all be creative, but we aren't. If you are not a creative person, you may surprise yourself by coming up with a great idea to make your life a little easier. This could be as simple as how you have your supplies set up at home to as complex as creating a daily plan that fits you personally.

You may think you don't have an ounce of creativity. Have you ever had a moment where everything clicked? A moment of discovery? An idea that you came up with? Creativity doesn't have to shout from art canvas or movie screens. It can be quiet inspirations we have throughout the day. Think of one of those

moments. How did it feel? How did you come to that moment?
Was there a process you could try again? Or can you take what
you learned from that and adapt it to your current situation?

Take a box of crayons. We are never too old to color a picture
and design whatever we want. As we grow, we lose that
childhood imagination and our thoughts get clouded by
reality. Tap into that childhood creativity and create a life you
love, even with diabetes. The following is a song I heard years
ago and never forgot it. It shows how others perspectives can
shape who we become, but we must remember that, as adults, we
can choose our own colors again.

Flowers Are Red

By Harry Chapin

The little boy went first day of school
He got some crayons and started to draw
He put colors all over the paper

Michelle A. Dart

For colors was what he saw
And the teacher said.. What you doin' young man
I'm paintin' flowers he said
She said... It's not the time for art young man
And anyway flowers are green and red

There's a time for everything young man

And a way it should be done
You've got to show concern for everyone else
For you're not the only one
And she said... Flowers are red

young man Green leaves are

green
There's no need to see flowers any other way
Than the way they always have been seen
But the little boy said...
There are so many colors in the rainbow
So many colors in the morning sun
So many colors in the flower and I see every one
Well the teacher said.. You're sassy
There's ways that things should be
And you'll paint flowers the way they are
So repeat after me.....

Diabetes Your Way

And she said... Flowers are red
young man Green Leaves are
green
There's no need to see flowers any other way
Than the way they always have been seen

But the little boy said...
There are so many colors in the rainbow
So many colors in the morning sun
So many colors in the flower and I see every one
The teacher put him in a corner
She said.. It's for your own good..
And you won't come out 'til you get it right
And are responding like you should Well
finally he got lonely
Frightened thoughts filled his head
And he went up to the teacher
And this is what he said.. and he said
Flowers are red, green leaves are green There's no
need to see flowers any other way Than the
way they always have been seen
Time went by like it always does
And they moved to another town And the
little boy went to another school And this
is what he found
But that little boy painted flowers

The teacher there was smilin' She
said...Painting should be fun
And there are so many colors in a
flower
So let's use every one In neat rows of
green and red And when the teacher
asked him why This is what he said.
And he said,
Flowers are red, green Leaves are green There's no
need to see flowers any other way Than the
way they always have been seen.

Just as there are many colors in a rainbow, there are many ways to manage diabetes successfully. Let your creativity color your life. It's okay to tap into other people's creativity. Learn about how others manage their diabetes. Talking with other people with diabetes can provide us with some excellent ideas that appeal to us and our lifestyles. Just because it is appealing, doesn't mean it is the best option, though. When trying new things, we must always be vigilant to how it impacts our life and our diabetes.

Don't give up if something doesn't work the first time. Some things will need tweaking to make it work for you. Where can you get ideas from other people? Local support groups can be a great place to learn how to deal with a variety of issues. Life with diabetes is more than thinking like a pancreas (although that helps, too!). Diabetes impacts our physical and emotional life. It can play a part in our relationships, our ability to work and turn our lives upside down. If approached with our toolbox in hand, we can protect ourselves from some of the challenges, but we can't predict the end result.

Brainstorming is another great way to come up with creative ideas. Write down every idea that comes to mind when you think of an issue. It doesn't have to make sense, write it down anyway. After you have written everything you can think of, look through your list. Find what speaks to you and explore it. You never know where it will take you. It may help you come up with answers you have been searching for.

Talk about it. Remember, we gain insight when we share our story with others. Their feedback may spark new ideas or you may find ideas come to you as you speak. Holding it in is like keeping your garden from sunlight and water. It will be very difficult to grow. Give yourself every opportunity to accomplish your goals.

Creativity can be nurtured in many ways. Keep tapping into it and you will find that it grows. Keep your mind open and active. Pay attention to your surroundings. There is inspiration everywhere.

Michelle A. Dart

Chapter 10 — The Reality of it All

The reality is that you have diabetes (just stating the obvious). The reality is that living healthy will improve the health of your body and decrease risks for complications. The reality is that a diagnosis of diabetes can significantly change your life (again, this is not new information). The reality is you do have choices. The reality is that you can live a life you love with diabetes.

It would be nice to live in a fantasy world where we all are healthy, happy and thriving. Real life can be a struggle and sometimes it is not the diabetes that is the source of the problem, but the diabetes is affected by those other issues. The reality is you are a whole person, who is not defined by having diabetes. It would be easy if diabetes were the only thing in life you had to worry about, but it's not. So, where does diabetes fit into your life?

Priorities shift. There is a lot of giving and taking, and many choices to make every day. You are in charge of how you live each day.

When you make a conscious decision to do a blood sugar test, you choose to learn more about your diabetes. It is valuable information that gives you clues that can help you see patterns that work or don't work. When you make a conscious decision to exercise your arms and legs while watching television, you choose to make every movement count. Every time you choose a healthier option, you are choosing to improve your health. Good for you! You don't have to develop an elaborate lifestyle plan to make a difference. The reality is you may already be doing many great things for you, your health and your diabetes.

Maybe you see different areas of your routine that need improvement. Some of you may not really have a routine at all. That is your routine. It is just variable or flexible. You know you want something different and, when you are ready to make a change, it is important to ask yourself what you realistically can do to take a step toward living your life your way. I choose to move to Maui because the warmth and sunshine would be good for my health. I can list goals I would want to achieve while I was there, but the reality is that there are too many barriers right now that I can't change that get in the way. My point is, be realistic. It is okay to stretch outside of your comfort zone, but don't lose reality. And just because something doesn't seem like a viable option now, doesn't mean it won't be the best answer somewhere down the road.

Another reality is that you are not alone. There are people all around you facing similar challenges, only you can't tell by looking at them. Sometimes it may seem that having diabetes is like walking around with a huge billboard sign, but in reality, others do not know your story unless you offer it to them. Diabetes is not visible, making it often misunderstood.

You can choose to keep your diabetes to yourself, but the reality is the world needs to be educated. Who better to educate others than you?

A sad reality is people with diabetes still face discrimination in schools and the work place. This will continue until people have a better understanding about Type 1 and Type 2 Diabetes, as well as the other forms of diabetes that we are hearing more about. There is latent onset autoimmune diabetes in adulthood and maturity onset diabetes of youth, to name a couple. It is a very complex illness that impacts every facet of our lives.

A positive reality is the technology to manage diabetes of all forms is improving. Could there be a cure someday? I believe it's possible. I look forward to that becoming reality. In the meantime, we have to make the best of what we have and those who are especially inspired may help us leap ahead toward a cure. Put on your oxygen mask first and create the life you love with successful diabetes management. Then you can move onto new ideas and new projects that will be stepping stones to great discoveries.

Whatever your reality is, it doesn't have to stay unchanged. We are so lucky to have the ability to change our reality. Our reality also can change without notice or through any control of our own. It is what we do with our reality that will determine where we go. Take the road you are comfortable with. If you need consistency and routine, take the well-paved road with set standards and follow them. You can get to the same end-point if you take the dirt path, but you have to put on your explorer hat and be willing to try new things. If you have an adventurous spirit, this may be just what you are looking for. Either road can have hills and valleys, bumps, roadblocks or even a washout. Life can be messy. Make the best of your reality and enjoy the view!

Michelle A. Dart

Chapter 11— Resource Guide

- American Diabetes Association — diabetes.org

   o 1-800-342-2383

- Juvenile Diabetes Research Foundation

   International — jdrf.org

   o 1-800-533-2873

- National Center for Chronic Disease Prevention and

   Health Promotion — cdc.gov/diabetes

   o 1-800-232-4636

- National Diabetes Education Program —

   ndep.nih.gov

   o 1-888-693-6337

- National Diabetes Information Clearinghouse —

   diabetes.niddk.nih.gov

   o 1-800-860-8747

   o 1-886-569-1162 TTY

Directory of Diabetes Organizations:

diabetes.niddk.nih.gov/resources/Directory_Diabetes_Or

gs_508.pdf

Information on diabetes-related complications:

- National Eye Institute -
  nei.nih.gov/health/diabetic/retinopathy.asp;

  1-301-496-5248

- American Chronic Pain Association - theacpa.org;
  1-800-533-3231

- National Institute of Neurological Disorders and
  Stroke - www.ninds.nih.gov; 1-800-352-9424

- National Kidney Foundation -
  kidney.org/atoz/atozTopic_Diabetes.cfm;

  1-800-622-9010

- American Heart Association - heart.org;

  1-800-242-8721

- Centers for Disease Control (CDC) -
  www.cdc.gov/diabetes; 1-800-232-4636

Local Resources

§ Ask your provider if there are any local support

groups, diabetes education programs, cooking

classes, resources for diabetes supplies

§ Check with local Lion's and Kiwanis clubs

§ Call your local health department and ask about any resources available

§ Your state department of health has resources available as well

§ Grocery stores often have a nutritionist available. Inquire if they provide supermarket tours

§ You can locate local certified diabetes educators through the American Association of Diabetes Educators (see next page)

§ There are diabetes coaching programs available online that can be provided by phone, email and even texting. Here are a couple options, but you can also do an online search:

 o darthealthcc.com

 o fit4d.com

§ Call your health insurance carrier and inquire if they have a diabetes coaching program staffed by certified diabetes educators

§   If you need support dealing with issues in schools with diabetes, your state health department may have a program that pays a diabetes educator to provide education to the schools.

§   Other school resources include:

o childrenwithdiabetes.com (parent

perspective, resources for management)

o jdrf.org (guidelines, advocacy)

o diabetes.org (Safe at School Program,

advocacy)

Diabetes Education

☐   diabeteseducator.org/DiabetesEducation/Find.html

☐   medicare.gov/coverage/diabetes- screenings.html

Financial Assistance

☐ diabetes.niddk.nih.gov/dm/pubs/financialhelp

☐ cdc.gov/diabetes/consumer/financial.htm

☐ isletsofhope.com/pdf/diabetes-assistance-

programs.pdf

☐ defeatdiabetes.org/self_management

☐ diabetes.org/living-with-diabetes/parents-and-

kids/ada-camps/financial-assistance.html

Pharmaceutical Companies

- Together Rx Access: togetherrxaccess.com
  - 1-800-444-4106
  - a collaboration including Abbott Laboratories,
    Bristol-Myers Squibb, GlaxoSmithKline, Johnson
    & Johnson, LifeScan, Novartis, Ortho Biotech,
    Pfizer, and Takeda Pharmaceuticals.

- Abbott Diabetes Care Patient Assistance Program:
  abbottpatientassistancefoundation.org
  - 1-800-222-6885

- Amylin Patient Assistance Program:
  amylin.com/products/patient-resources/patient-
  assistance-program.htm
  - 1-800-330-7647

- AstraZeneca Foundation Patient Assistance Program: astrazeneca-us.com/help-affording- your-medicines
  - 1-800-292-6363

- Bayer Patient Assistance Program:
  - 1-800-998-9180

- Bristol-Myers Squibb Patient Assistance Foundation: bmspaf.org
  - 1-800-736-0003

- Eli Lilly and Company's Lilly Cares: lillycares.com
  - 1-800-545-6962

- GlaxoSmithKline's Patient Assistance Programs: gskforyou.com
  - 1-866-728-4368

- Johnson & Johnson's Access2Wellness Program: access2wellness.com
  - 1-800-652-6227

- Merck Patient Assistance Program merck.com/merckhelps
  - 1-800-994-2111

- Merck/Sherling-Plough Patient Assistance Program: msppharma.com/msp_jv/msppharma/patient_assist
  - 1-800-347-7503

- Novartis Patient Assistance Foundation: pharma.us.novartis.com/about-us/our-patient-caregiver-resources/paf-enrollment.jsp
  - 1-800-277-2254

- Novo Nordisk Diabetes Patient Assistance Program: levemir-us.com/paying-patient-assistance.asp
  - 1-866-310-7549

- Pfizer Helpful Answers: pfizerhelpfulanswers.com
  - 1-800-706-2400

- Pfizer Bridge Program: genotropin.com/content/Support_center_pfizer_bridge_program.aspx
  - 1-800-645-1280

- Roche ACCU-CHEK Patient Assistance Programs: accu-chek.com/us/customer-care/patient-assistance-program.html
  - 1-877-757-6243

- Sanofi-Aventis Patient Assistance Program: sanofi- aventis.us
  - 1-800-221-4025

- Schering-Plough Patient Assistance Program: schering-plough.com/products/patient-assistance.aspx
  - 1-800-656-9485

- Takeda Patient Assistance Program:
  tpna.com/responsibility/patient_assistance_
  program.aspx
  - 1-800-830-9159

Mail Order Companies

- Ordering via mail can save you money. Call your
  insurance carrier to determine the best mail order
  company for you.

Blogs
- empowered2bme.wordpress.com

- diabetesdaily.com

- diabetesmine.com

- diabetesselfmanagement.com/blog

- sixuntilme.com

- scottsdiabetes.com

Michelle A. Dart

Chapter 12 – For the Parents and Caregivers

The support you provide is invaluable. You may not get praise
every day for all that you do, but you are making a difference.
Much of the information in this book can be helpful for you in
your support role. You are riding the roller coaster of diabetes
right along with your loved one because you are emotionally
invested.

Being a support person is very difficult. We only want the best
for them. Information about diabetes comes at us from all
directions. We read about it in the newspaper, see it on
television and hear from other people about the "right" way
to live with diabetes. All of this information shapes our
perception. Remember, your loved one is unique and can't be
found in a textbook.

Interactions with our loved ones are directly impacted by what
we believe to be true. We want to see our children grow to make

healthy choices. They learn by watching us, clearly influencing their future decisions. We want our parent to take better care of himself or herself so we can keep them around longer or prevent them from suffering complications. We feel helpless. Instinct is to try to fix what we perceive to be a problem.

Loved ones ultimately choose to live their life in their own way. How can we deal with this when we see they are making "poor" decisions? Do they have enough understanding to be able to make a decision and understand the consequences? If they don't fully understand, help them. Often times, our loved ones do not learn as well when we try to explain things that we understand to be true. A diabetes educator that works with a coaching perspective can help. This person can help them better understand their diabetes and how their choices impact their life.

Support people need education as well. Information and recommendations for diabetes management change often, so it is important to stay up to date so we don't add to misinformation the person with diabetes may already have.

In order to be the best support person you can be, stay

educated.

Parenting a child with diabetes has its own challenges. An entire

family changes with this diagnosis. The child with diabetes

needs to be monitored closely, yet needs to be able to be a kid.

We are pulled to protect them from any harm and quickly learn

to advocate for our child. We need to be well educated, not only

to safely care for our child, but so we can educate others. We

depend on childcare and school to keep our children safe, yet

allow them to be a kid. How do we protect them when they are

not with us? Education! See Chapter 11 for resources related to

children with diabetes.

We know our child best. We see what works and what doesn't.

We are responsible for teaching them how to manage their

diabetes as they become developmentally ready for different

aspects of their care. This information is needed when

working with your child's health care provider. You are a team raising a captain.

If your loved one is an adult this can be frustrating. Are they being stubborn or are they exercising their right to make educated decisions? Encourage your loved one to stay up on diabetes education as recommendations change and may improve their life. Look at the big picture. How much control does your loved one have over their current lifestyle? Fixed income can make it difficult to afford healthy foods and disabilities interfere with the amount of exercise performed. Age brings about many physical issues that interfere with our loved ones always keeping up with a healthy lifestyle. Vision changes may keep someone from moving around because of the fear of falling. Pain can make it almost impossible to walk. Decreased appetites increase the risk of low blood sugars.

Many adults do not realize they can learn to manage their diabetes and make choices of their own. It wasn't very long ago that people started being more involved instead of waiting for the

doctor to tell them what to do. The adult with diabetes may be used

to getting direction from the health care provider and never do

anything without consulting the provider. This is dictated by their

comfort level. The best role you can take is that of standing beside

them, helping to educate them and empowering them to make the

best decisions for them.

This does not mean that a person who is neglecting their diabetes

and putting their life at risk gets praised for taking charge. This

needs to be addressed. Neglect can be a sign of depression, which is

common with diabetes. It's time for an exploration to find out

what is keeping them from making better choices.

Chances are you will not always agree with the way your loved one

cares for himself. Learning why they make the choices they do is

just as important as exploring your reasons for disagreeing. That

information may be helpful to them or may at least open doors to

more conversations that empower them to make better choices.

Michelle A. Dart

Chapter 13 — 15 Minutes a Day
to Better Diabetes Control

1. You can test your blood sugar 3-5x/day or more!

2. It takes approximately 15 minutes to prepare and take oral diabetes medications 2-3x/day.

3. It takes <15 minutes to prepare and take insulin injections 4x/day

4. You can examine your injection sites or pump sites for any lumps, bruising, redness or tenderness in <15 minutes.

5. Safely treat a low blood sugar. Remember 15 grams of carbohydrates and retest 15 minutes later!

6. Reasonably be able to decrease a high blood sugar through use of insulin (only as advised by your healthcare provider), exercise (as long as there are no ketones. Follow what your healthcare provider recommends), fluids (water is helpful, but not a solution alone) or rest (if related to adrenaline from exercise or stress).

7.   This could be a full exercise routine! – You would be

      amazed by the amount of activity you can do in

      15 minutes! Time yourself. You don't have to run a

      marathon, any movement will do.

8.   Create a healthy menu for meals this week and a

      grocery list so you have everything you need!

9.   Create a new goal.

10.   Develop a plan to accomplish your goal.

11.   Review your blood sugar readings and track patterns.

      Your diabetes educator can help with this if you aren't

      comfortable.

12.   Meditate or do something to decrease stress. Stress has a

      significant impact on our blood sugars.

13.   Cat Nap-I'm not saying take a three-hour nap every

      day, but listen to your body when it is tired. Good sleep

      has a lot to do with healthy blood sugars and overall

      diabetes control.

14. Tell your story- this can be inspiring and motivating, not

    only to you, but to everyone who reads it. Send your

    stories to shareyourstory@ringopub.com

15. Reward yourself for being amazing!

Share Your Story!

I was serious when I encouraged you to share your story with me, anyone, or everyone. You can share your story anonymously if you want. You can choose whether or not you want it published in a book of compiled stories about true life with diabetes. Stories should be real and honest about the challenges and triumphs that come with living with diabetes.

Your story may be just the story to inspire someone who is struggling with diabetes. Empowering other people can empower us as well. Send your stories to:

shareyourstory@ringopub.com

Ringo Publishing, Inc.

Share Your Story

PO Box 180

Skaneateles, NY 13152

Thank you for sharing a part of your life. If you have suggestions for a charitable organization that could benefit from the sales of the "Share Your Stories" series, please send them with your submission. Recommendations for a charitable organization to benefit from a portion of proceeds from our booksales is needed!

Your opinion is welcome!

Please send all comments and reviews to

customerservice@ringopub.com or

Ringo Publishing, Inc.

Diabetes Your Way

PO Box 180

Skaneateles, NY 13152

**Bulk orders are available at special pricing!

Send an inquiry with any comments, suggestions or

reviews.

Watch for more books that will benefit diabetes research and

programs. If you know a child with Type 1 Diabetes, check out

"Danny, the Diabetes Dynamo." This book provides

donations to the American Diabetes Association and the Juvenile

Diabetes Research Foundation. This is the beginning of a series

of children's books that aim to promote self-management

according to developmental stage.

Michelle A. Dart

About the Author

Michelle A. Dart holds a master's degree in nursing and has worked as a pediatric nurse practitioner in Upstate New York. In 1995, she graduated from Elmira College with a bachelor's degree in nursing and obtained a master's degree in 2001 through Upstate Medical University. While working with children with diabetes and their families, she became a certified diabetes educator and has been the facilitator of a diabetes support group sponsored by a local community health organization for the past several years.

Michelle has authored "Motivational Interviewing in Nursing Practice: Empowering the Patient," a nursing textbook about a way of communicating that promotes behavior change. In 2010, Michelle self-published the book entitled "Danny, the Diabetes Dynamo," a book for children newly diagnosed or early in their diagnosis of Type 1 Diabetes. This book is the beginning of a series to help children learn self-management skills. A portion of the proceeds are donated to the American Diabetes Association and the Juvenile Diabetes Research Foundation.

Michelle is a member of the American Association of Diabetes Educators, the American Diabetes Association, the Obesity Society, the Obesity Action Coalition, the Diabetes

Education and Camping Association and the American Camping Association. In addition, she is a member of the National Association of Professional Women. She is on the review committee for the development of professional standards of practice for nurse health coaching. Michelle provides diabetes education in school and daycare settings as a consultant with the New York State Department of Health.

In early 2012, Michelle founded Dart Health Coaching & Consulting to provide coaching to people affected by diabetes, including but not limited to those with Type 1 and Type 2 Diabetes, parents of children with diabetes, adolescents/young adults with diabetes and support persons. Consulting services are provided in areas of Motivational Interviewing, health coaching, and diabetes education. She is available for coaching services, consulting and speaking engagements.

Michelle lives in Auburn, NY, with her husband and three children. She has a son with Type 1 Diabetes and a parent with Type 2 Diabetes. This has provided her with her most valuable experiences to motivate her to contribute to the diabetes community.

Diabetes Your Way

Please feel free to use the following pages to make notes to yourself, to brainstorm or write out your goals and plans to achieve them. The pages are blank so you can create what you want with as many colors as you would like. Write about your story. Most of all create a life you love and live with Diabetes Your Way!

Michelle A. Dart